Diverticulitis

Listed Common treatment functions that would help diverticulitis patients

Dr Walt wade

Contents

Chapter1

Introduction to diverticultis

Diverticulitis is a commonly diagnosed medical condition that affects the colon. It is characterized by the inflammation or infection of small pockets in the colon wall, known as diverticula. These pockets can develop when weak spots in the colon's inner lining bulge outward and become filled with feces. The condition is often asymptomatic, meaning many individuals may not even be aware that they have diverticulitis. However, in more severe cases, it can cause digestive issues and lead to complications that require medical treatment. The prevalence of diverticulitis is gradually increasing worldwide, with more developed countries being impacted the most. It is primarily a disease of the elderly, with the majority of cases being diagnosed in individuals over the age of 40. However, it can also occur in younger adults, especially those who have weakened colon walls due to genetic predisposition or lifestyle factors. Diverticulitis is linked to several risk factors, the most prominent being a low-fiber diet. A diet lacking in fiber can cause the stool to become hard and dense, making it harder to pass through the colon and leading to increased pressure on the colon walls. This pressure can cause diverticula to form and become inflamed or infected. Other risk factors include obesity, lack of physical activity, smoking, and a family history of the disease. The exact cause of diverticulitis is still unknown. However, researchers believe that genetics, lifestyle, and diet all play significant roles in its development. Studies have shown that individuals with connective tissue disorders, such as Ehlers-Danlos syndrome and Marfan syndrome, are more likely to develop diverticulitis. Additionally, a diet high in red meat and low in fruits, vegetables, and whole grains is also associated with a higher risk of developing the condition. Diverticulitis is a progressive disease, meaning that it can develop in stages, starting with a condition known as diverticulosis. Diverticulosis is the formation of small, pouch-like pockets in the colon wall that do not cause any symptoms. However, as these pockets increase in number and size, they can become inflamed or infected, leading to diverticulitis. The severity of diverticulitis can vary, ranging from mild cases that can be treated with simple dietary changes to severe cases that require hospitalization and surgical intervention. The most common symptoms associated with diverticulitis include abdominal pain, bloating, constipation, and diarrhea. These symptoms can be caused by inflammation or infection in the diverticula, and they can range from mild to severe. In some cases, the inflammation can be confined to a small area and cause localized pain. In other cases, the entire colon may be affected, causing severe pain, fever, and chills. Additionally, complications such as abscesses, bleeding, and bowel obstruction can occur in severe cases of diverticulitis. To diagnose diverticulitis, a doctor will typically perform a physical exam and obtain a detailed medical history. They may also recommend diagnostic tests such as a CT scan or a colonoscopy to confirm the presence of diverticula and check for any signs of inflammation or infection. Blood tests may also be conducted to check for any abnormalities or signs of infection. Diverticulitis is a treatable condition, and in most cases, it can be managed with lifestyle changes and medications. The treatment plan will depend on the severity of the condition and the presence of any complications. Mild cases of diverticulitis can be managed at home with a clear liquid diet, antibiotics, and pain relievers. However, more severe cases may require hospitalization, intravenous antibiotics, and, in some cases, surgical intervention. Surgery for diverticulitis is typically recommended for individuals who do not respond to conservative treatment methods or for those who experience recurrent episodes of the condition. The most common surgery for diverticulitis is a colectomy, which involves the removal of the affected part of the colon. In some cases, a temporary colostomy may also be required to allow the colon to heal properly. Prevention of diverticulitis is centered around maintaining a healthy diet and lifestyle. Eating a diet rich in fiber, including fruits, vegetables, and whole grains, can help prevent the formation of diverticula. It is also essential to stay hydrated, maintain a healthy weight, and exercise regularly to keep the colon functioning correctly. Additionally, smoking should be avoided, as it can increase the risk of developing diverticulitis. In conclusion, diverticulitis is a common condition that affects the colon and is linked to multiple risk factors, including age, diet, and lifestyle. While it can be asymptomatic, it can also cause uncomfortable symptoms and lead to serious complications. It is essential to understand the underlying causes and take preventative measures, such as maintaining a healthy diet and lifestyle, to reduce the risk of developing this condition. With proper treatment and management, individuals with diverticulitis can lead a healthy and comfortable life.

chapter2

diverticultis treatment

Treatment for diverticulitis typically depends on the severity and frequency of symptoms, as well as the individual's medical history. Here are some common treatment options for diverticulitis: 1. Antibiotics: If the diverticulitis is not severe, the doctor may prescribe antibiotics to treat the infection and reduce inflammation. The type and duration of antibiotics will depend on the severity of the infection and the person's overall health. Antibiotics may also be prescribed after surgery to prevent infections. 2. Pain relievers: Diverticulitis can cause abdominal pain, which can be managed with over-the-counter or prescription pain medications. Nonsteroidal anti-inflammatory drugs (NSAIDs) such as ibuprofen or acetaminophen may help relieve mild pain, while more severe pain may require prescription medication. 3. Clear liquid diet: During a diverticulitis flare-up, the doctor may recommend a clear liquid diet for a few days to give the digestive system a break and allow the inflammation to subside. Clear liquids like broth, water, and juice can provide essential nutrients while being easy to digest. 4. High-fiber diet: Once the diverticulitis has resolved, the doctor may recommend a high-fiber diet to promote regular bowel movements and prevent future episodes. Foods high in fiber, such as fruits, vegetables, whole grains, and legumes, can help soften stools and promote bowel movement regularity. 5. Fiber supplements: If it is difficult to consume enough fiber through diet alone, the doctor may recommend a fiber supplement. These supplements come in various forms, such as powders, pills, or chewable tablets, and can help increase fiber intake to prevent constipation and reduce pressure on the diverticula. 6. Probiotics: Probiotics are live bacteria and yeasts that are beneficial for digestive health. They can help restore the balance of good bacteria in the gut and may ease symptoms of diverticulitis. Probiotics can be found in supplements or foods such as yogurt, kefir, and sauerkraut. 7. Surgery: In severe cases or if complications arise, surgery may be necessary. The most common surgery for diverticulitis is a colon resection, in which the affected portion of the large intestine is removed and the remaining ends are reconnected. Surgery is typically only recommended if the person has had multiple episodes of diverticulitis or has complications such as abscesses, fistulae, or scarring of the intestine. In addition to these treatment options, there are several self-care measures that individuals with diverticulitis can take to manage their symptoms and prevent future episodes. These include: 1. Drink plenty of fluids: Staying hydrated is important for keeping stools soft and preventing constipation. In addition, adequate hydration can help flush out any toxins or bacteria that may be contributing to the infection. 2. Exercise regularly: Regular exercise can help promote regular bowel movements and keep the digestive system functioning properly. 3. Avoid foods that can aggravate diverticulitis: Foods that are hard to digest, such as nuts, seeds, and popcorn, can irritate the diverticula and should be avoided during a flare-up. Spicy foods or foods high in fat or refined sugar may also cause discomfort and should be limited. 4. Quit smoking: Smoking can contribute to inflammation in the digestive tract and can increase the risk of complications from diverticulitis. Quitting smoking can help improve overall health and reduce the risk of future episodes. 5. Manage stress: Stress can worsen symptoms of diverticulitis.

Learning stress management techniques, such as deep breathing, meditation, or yoga, can help promote relaxation and reduce the impact of stress on the body. It is crucial for individuals with diverticulitis to follow their doctor's recommendations and make lifestyle changes to manage their condition. If left untreated, diverticulitis can lead to serious complications that may require hospitalization or surgery. By following these treatment and self-care measures, individuals can successfully manage their symptoms and prevent future episodes of diverticulitis. In addition to medical treatments, there are also alternative therapies that may help reduce symptoms and prevent recurrent episodes of diverticulitis. These include: 1. Acupuncture: This ancient Chinese practice involves inserting thin needles into specific points on the body. Acupuncture has been used to treat a variety of digestive disorders, including diverticulitis. 2. Herbal supplements: Some herbs, such as aloe vera, flaxseed, and slippery elm, can help ease digestive symptoms and promote regular bowel movements. However, it is important to consult a healthcare professional before taking any herbal supplements as they may interact with other medications or have side effects. 3. Probiotic enemas: Probiotic enemas involve inserting a liquid solution containing probiotics into the rectum. This therapy aims to introduce good bacteria directly into the gut to help restore the balance of the intestinal microbiome. While these alternative therapies may provide relief for some individuals, they should not be used as a replacement for medical treatment and should be discussed with a healthcare professional before trying.

chapter3

diverticultis diet

The primary goal of a diverticulitis diet is to reduce inflammation and allow the digestive tract to rest and heal. It involves making changes to your eating habits and incorporating foods that are easy to digest and provide the necessary nutrients for proper healing. Below, we will discuss in detail the aspects of a diverticulitis diet and the foods recommended for this condition. What to Eat One of the key components of a diverticulitis diet is to increase the intake of fiber. This is because a high fiber diet promotes regular bowel movements and helps prevent constipation, which can put strain on the colon and cause diverticula to form.

Additionally, fiber aids in keeping the digestive tract healthy and prevents the formation of new diverticula. The recommended daily intake of fiber for adults is 25-30 grams, but this may vary based on individual needs. When choosing high fiber foods, it is important to focus on the type of fiber as well. There are two types of fiber: soluble and insoluble. Soluble fiber, found in foods like oats, beans, and apples, helps soften stools and makes them easier to pass. Insoluble fiber, found in foods like whole grains, nuts, and vegetables, adds bulk to stool and helps move it more efficiently through the digestive tract. A healthy diverticulitis diet should include a variety of foods that provide both types of fiber. Another important aspect of a diverticulitis diet is to increase the intake of fluids. Adequate hydration helps prevent constipation and keeps stools soft, making them easier to pass. Water is the best choice, but other options like herbal teas, broths, and fresh juices can also contribute to daily fluid intake. In addition to increasing fiber and fluid intake, there are certain foods that are recommended for a diverticulitis diet. These include: 1. High-fiber fruits and vegetables - These include fruits like apples, bananas, and berries, as well as vegetables like broccoli, carrots, and squash. Fresh, frozen, or canned versions are all acceptable, but it is important to avoid fruits and vegetables that are high in small seeds, such as strawberries or tomatoes, as they may get stuck in the pouches and cause discomfort. 2. Whole grains - Whole wheat bread, brown rice, and whole grain pastas are all good sources of fiber. These should be consumed in moderation, as too much can cause bloating or gas. 3. Lean proteins - Healthy protein sources, like chicken, fish, tofu, and eggs, should be included in a diverticulitis diet. These foods are also easy to digest and can help provide necessary nutrients for the body to heal. 4. Low-fat dairy - Dairy products, like yogurt, cheese, and milk, should be chosen in low-fat or non-fat versions to reduce the intake of saturated fats. These products are also good sources of calcium, which can be beneficial for overall health. 5. Healthy oils - Olive, canola, and flaxseed oils are rich in omega-3 fatty acids, which have anti-inflammatory properties and can help reduce symptoms of diverticulitis. However, these should be used in moderation, as excessive intake can lead to diarrhea. What to Avoid On the other hand, there are certain foods that should be avoided or consumed in limited amounts when following a diverticulitis diet. These include: 1. Red meat - High intake of red meat, including beef, pork, and lamb, has been linked to an increased risk of diverticulitis. It is recommended to limit red meat intake and choose leaner cuts when consuming it. 2. Highly processed foods - Foods like chips, cookies, and other snack foods are typically low in fiber and high in unhealthy fats and sugars. These should be avoided as part of a diverticulitis diet. 3. Spicy foods - Spicy foods can irritate the digestive tract and increase symptoms in people with diverticulitis. It is best to avoid or limit spicy foods in your diet. 4. Foods high in added sugars - Foods like soda, candy, and other sweets should be consumed in moderation or avoided completely. These foods can cause bloating, gas, and discomfort in people with diverticulitis. 5. Seeds and nuts - While seeds and nuts are generally considered healthy, they can get lodged in the diverticula and cause discomfort. If you do choose to consume these foods, it is best to grind or puree them first. Meal Ideas It can be challenging to come up with meal ideas when following a diverticulitis diet. Here are a few simple and delicious meals that you can incorporate into your diet: 1. Oatmeal with fresh berries and almond butter. 2. Grilled chicken with quinoa and steamed vegetables. 3. Fish tacos with whole wheat tortillas, black beans, and avocado. 4. Spinach and chicken salad with a light vinaigrette dressing. 5. Whole wheat pasta with tomato sauce, lean ground turkey, and sautéed vegetables. 6. Baked sweet potato with steamed broccoli and grilled salmon. 7. Vegetable and bean chili with a side of whole grain crackers. It is important to note that everyone's dietary needs are different, and it is always best to consult with a healthcare professional before making any major dietary changes. Additionally, keeping a food journal can be helpful in tracking what foods trigger symptoms and which ones are well-tolerated.

diverticultis causes

One of the primary causes of diverticulitis is a low-fiber diet. The Western diet, which is high in processed foods, red meat, and saturated fats, is associated with a higher risk of diverticulitis. A low-fiber diet can lead to constipation, which increases the pressure on the colon wall, causing the formation of pouches. When these pouches become inflamed or infected, they can cause diverticulitis. A diet that is low in fiber can also lead to a lack of stool bulk, which can result in hard, difficult-to-pass stools. As a result, the colon must work harder to eliminate waste, potentially leading to increased pressure on the colon wall and diverticula formation. Another contributing factor to diverticulitis is age. As people age, the walls of their colon weaken, making them more susceptible to the formation of diverticula. The majority of people diagnosed with diverticulitis are over the age of 60. This is partly due to the weakening of the muscle walls, making it more difficult for the colon to contract and move waste through the digestive system effectively. Age-related changes in the digestive tract, such as decreased blood flow and decreased nerve function, may also contribute to diverticula formation. Obesity is also linked to an increased risk of diverticulitis. Excess body weight puts added pressure on the colon, increasing the likelihood of diverticula formation. Furthermore, obesity is often accompanied by a high-fat, low-fiber diet, which can further exacerbate the risk of diverticulitis. Studies have shown that individuals with a body mass index (BMI) of 30 or higher have a higher risk of developing diverticulitis compared to those with a healthy BMI. Another potential cause of diverticulitis is the use of nonsteroidal anti-inflammatory drugs (NSAIDs). These medications, such as aspirin and ibuprofen, are commonly used to manage pain and inflammation. However, they can irritate the lining of the digestive tract, increasing the risk of diverticulitis. A study published in the American Journal of Gastroenterology found that individuals who regularly used NSAIDs were more likely to develop diverticulitis than those who did not use these medications. Genetics is also believed to play a role in the development of diverticulitis. While specific genes and genetic mutations have not been identified, studies have shown that individuals with a family history of diverticulitis have a higher risk of developing the condition. This suggests that genetics may predispose individuals to diverticula formation, making them more susceptible to developing diverticulitis. Smoking has also been linked to an increased risk of diverticulitis. Smoking can lead to decreased blood flow and damage to the lining of the colon, which can contribute to the formation of diverticula. Furthermore, smoking has been shown to weaken the immune system, making individuals more susceptible to infections, including diverticulitis. Various medical conditions can also contribute to diverticulitis. These include inflammatory bowel diseases (IBD) such as Crohn's disease and ulcerative colitis. In these conditions, inflammation can damage the lining of the colon, leading to the formation of diverticula. Diverticulitis is also more common in individuals with a weakened immune system, such as those with HIV/AIDS or undergoing chemotherapy. In rare cases, diverticulitis may be caused by physical obstructions in the colon, such as scars or narrowing of the colon, which can cause increased pressure in the area. Other possible causes of diverticulitis include a lack of physical activity, prior episodes of diverticulitis, and a diet high in red meat.

chapter4

diverticultis symptoms female

The most common symptom of diverticulitis in women is abdominal pain. This pain can range from mild to severe and is often described as cramping or sharp in nature. Women may experience this pain in the lower left side of the abdomen, but it can also be felt in other areas, such as the right side or even the entire abdomen. The pain may worsen after eating, and can also be accompanied by bloating, gas, and nausea. Another common symptom of diverticulitis in females is changes in bowel habits. Women may experience constipation or diarrhea, as well as alternating between the two. This can be very uncomfortable and disruptive to daily routines. In severe cases, there may be blood in the stool. It is important to note that these changes in bowel habits can also be caused by other conditions, so it is crucial to consult a doctor for a proper diagnosis. Fever and chills are also commonly reported symptoms of diverticulitis in women. This is a result of the body's immune response to the inflammation or infection in the colon. The fever may be low-grade or high, and can come and go throughout the day. It is important to monitor the fever closely and consult a doctor if it persists or becomes particularly high. In some cases, women with diverticulitis may experience urinary symptoms. This can include frequent urination, urgency, and pain or discomfort while urinating. These symptoms can be a result of the inflamed sigmoid colon pressing on the bladder, causing irritation. It is important to note that these symptoms can also indicate a urinary tract infection, which can be a serious condition if left untreated. Fatigue and lack of energy are also common symptoms among women with diverticulitis. This is a result of the body being in a constant state of inflammation and infection, which can cause the body to feel drained and weak. This can greatly impact a woman's ability to carry out daily tasks and can lead to feelings of frustration and helplessness. Perhaps one of the most distressing symptoms of diverticulitis in females is pelvic pain. This pain may be constant or intermittent and can be sharp or dull in nature. It can also radiate to other areas, such as the lower back or thighs. The pelvic pain can be particularly difficult to manage, as it can greatly impact a woman's ability to move and carry out daily activities. In some cases, it may interfere with sexual intercourse, leading to a strain on intimate relationships. In severe cases of diverticulitis, women may experience complications such as abscesses or fistulas. An abscess occurs when the infection in the colon forms a pocket of pus, which can lead to intense, localized pain. A fistula is a more serious complication, where an abnormal passageway forms between different organs or tissues. This can lead to a range of symptoms, such as vaginal discharge, bowel obstruction, and severe pain. It is important to note that the symptoms of diverticulitis in females can vary greatly and may not necessarily present with all of the aforementioned symptoms. Some women may only experience one or two symptoms, while others may have a cluster of symptoms that greatly impact their daily lives. Therefore, it is crucial to pay attention to your body and seek medical attention if you experience any concerning changes or discomfort. The exact cause of diverticulitis is not fully understood, but there are several risk factors that have been identified. Age is a significant risk factor, as the prevalence of diverticulitis increases with age. Other risk factors include a diet low in fiber, obesity, physical inactivity, smoking, and certain medications such as NSAIDs. Diagnosing diverticulitis in females can be challenging, as the symptoms can be similar to other conditions such as irritable bowel syndrome or ovarian cysts. A physical examination, along with imaging tests such as an abdominal ultrasound or CT scan, can help to confirm a diagnosis. Blood tests may also be used to check for inflammation and infection in the body. Treatment for diverticulitis may involve a combination of medication and lifestyle changes. Antibiotics are often prescribed to help eliminate the infection, and pain relievers may be used to alleviate discomfort. A low-fiber diet may be recommended initially, followed by a gradual increase in fiber intake as symptoms improve. In some cases, surgery may be necessary to remove the affected colon or repair any complications.

The end